15 Minutes Daniel Fast Cookbook

Breakfast, Lunch, Appetizers, Dips, Seasoning, Lunch and Dinner Recipes

Disclaimer

What You Will Find In This Book?

If you are tired of eating takeout but between your work and family you do not have enough time to focus on cooking a meal for an hour or so, *50 Daniel Fast Recipes in 15 Minutes or Less* can definitely prove to be a lifesaver.

Processed foods are convenient and take less time to buy but they just are not the healthy option one looks for; after all you want the best for yourself. It's not as much about treating yourself as it is about taking care of yourself by engaging in a homemade healthy diet and that too by the renowned Daniel Fast.

And who does not want to impress their friends and loved ones with some quick cooking that will leave them awed. It all goes under the tag line that makes people say "how do they do it!"

The *50 Daniel Fast Recipes in 15 Minutes or Less* recipe book includes:
1. Authentic Daniel Fast less than 15 minute recipes, some even going down to 4 minutes.

2. A Range of High Protein breakfast cereals.

3. Recipes for dips and appetizers.

4. Cooking time, serving size and nutritional facts along with every recipe.

Just flip through the upcoming pages and look out for lots of healthy and time saving recipes.

Contents

Breakfast

Baked Apples or Pears

Serves 1
Nutritional Value: Calories: 9, Potassium: 7mg, Total Carbohydrates: 2.2g, Sugars: 2 g

Prep Time: 3 minutes

Cooking Time: 10 minutes

Ingredients
1 Pear/ Apple
½ teaspoon pure maple syrup
Crushed Cinnamon

Cooking Method
First cut the fruit, Apple or pear in half. Do not leave the center portion including the seeds in the fruit. Use a grape fruit spoon to scoop them out. You will specifically need a glass baking dish to bake the two halves of the fruit, which need to be placed skin side down on the glass, while you brush the top with maple syrup and sprinkle a dash of crushed cinnamon. Finally you can microwave the dish for 10 minutes and serve while warm.

Fruit and Nuts Granola

Serves 2
Nutritional Value: Total Fat: 55.2g, Sodium: 26mg, Potassium: 1430mg, Total Carbohydrates: 125.4 g, Protein: 36.7g.

Prep Time: 8 minutes

Cooking Time: 2 minutes

Ingredients
1 cup raisins
1 Tablespoon cinnamon
¼ cup flax seed
½ cup chopped walnuts
½ cup chopped cashews
½ cup unsalted sunflower seeds
½ cup chopped dry figs
½ cup slivered almonds
½ cup chopped unsweetened apricots (sweetened will do too)
A dash of chopped coconut
2.5 cups Oatmeal

Cooking Method
Use a large bowl to unload all the ingredients in and mix. Chop the fruits and nuts in a food blender separately (you can add them to the rest of the ingredients at the time of serving in the end a dash of cinnamon on top). Store the mixture in a tightly sealed container in an area of around 30oC. Prepare with unsweetened soy milk or water in the microwave to serve warm. To serve cold put ½ cup granola in soy milk and serve.

Muesli

Serves 1

Nutritional Value: Sodium: 7mg, Potassium: 2mg, Calcium: 1% Total Fat: 0.0g

Prep Time: 0 minutes

Cooking Time: 5 minutes

Ingredients
1 cup Muesli
1 cup water

Cooking Method
Boil water and add Muesli. Simmer for 5 minutes.

Oats, Apple and Blueberry Cereal

Serves 2

Nutritional Value: Calories: 895, Total Fat: 2.5g, Sodium 16 mg, Total Carbohydrates: 152.1g, Protein: 19.4g

Prep Time: 0 minutes

Cooking Time: 15 minutes

Ingredients

4 sweet apples
1 ½ cup rolled oats
2 cups blueberries
1 cup almonds
2 cups apple juice

Cooking Method

Chop the apples, grind the almonds and mix together. Cook the oats and the blueberries once cooked. Squirt a bit of apple juice and sprinkle the cereal with a dash of cinnamon and nutmeg.

Sweet Honey Cereal

Serves 1

Nutritional Value: Calories: 221, Total Fat: 4.8g, Total Carbohydrates: 35.4g, Protein: 9.4g

Prep Time: 0 minutes

Cooking Time: 10 minutes

Ingredients
1/2 cup Oatmeal
1/2 cup Soymilk or Water
Honey or a dash of Cinnamon

Cooking Method
Cook Oatmeal and prepare in milk or water. Serve with sprinkling cinnamon or a bit of honey.

Early Morning Fruit Smoothie

Serves 2

Nutritional Value: Calories: 206, Total Fat: 2.8g, Total Carbohydrates: 43.2g, Protein: 5.8g

Prep Time: 0 minutes

Cooking Time: 2 minutes

Ingredients
2 bananas
1 cup soy milk
1 cup frozen berries

Cooking Method
Stuff all ingredients into a food processor and blend until smooth. To boost the protein in your diet you can always add silken tofu.

Stir Fry Breakfast for a High Protein Diet

Serves 1

Nutritional Value: Calories: 60, Total Fat: 7.0g, Total Carbohydrates: 0.0g.-

Prep Time: 0 minutes

Cooking Time: 4 minutes

Ingredients
Sliced ½ onion
Chopped ¼ green pepper
½ tablespoon olive oil
½ cup sturdy tofu, cut in bits
Italian herbs

Cooking Method
First stir fry onions and green peppers for 2 to 3 minutes in a bit of olive oil. Toss in Italian herbs and tofu and turn off the heat when the vegetables go soft.

Banana Cereal

Serves 2

Nutritional Value: Calories: 158.6, Total Fat: 3.1g, Total Carbohydrates: 34.2g, Protein: 2.5g

Prep Time: 2 minutes

Cooking Time: 0 minutes

Ingredients

1 teaspoon flake coconut
¼ cup chopped fig
¼ cup dates, dried
¼ cup chopped apricot
1 tablespoon chopped almonds
1/3 cup blueberries
1 banana sliced

Cooking Method

Toss all ingredients in a bowl and pour milk.

Fruit and Veggie Smoothie

Serves 2

Nutritional Value: Calories: 91, Total Fat: 0.4g, Total Carbohydrates: 23.1g, Protein: 1.5g

Prep Time: 2 minutes

Cooking Time: 2 minutes

Ingredients
½ cup coconut water
½ cup pineapple chunks
½ cup ice
1 cup banana
1 cup baby spinach

Cooking Method
Toss all ingredients in blender and blend till smooth.

Scrambled Tofu

Serves 1

Nutritional Value: Calories: 105, Total Fat: 0.8g, Total Carbohydrates: 21.9g, Protein: 4.3g

Prep Time: 2 minutes

Cooking Time: 7 minutes

Ingredients
1 clove minced garlic
2 sliced green onions
1 diced red bell pepper
1 tablespoon minced fresh cilantro
1 box of firm tofu
½ diced onion
1 diced tomato
1 small diced zucchini
A dash of salt and pepper/tomato paste

Cooking Method
Brush pan with olive oil and toss all ingredients into the pan until the vegetables are soft. Sprinkle with salt and pepper or you can always add a bit of tomato paste if you like. Serve while hot.

Fruity Oats Porridge

Serves 2

Nutritional Value: Calories: 54, Total Fat: 0.1g, Total Carbohydrates: 14.4g, Protein: 0.6g

Prep Time: 2 minutes

Cooking Time: 7 minutes

Ingredients
2 cups water
¾ cup oats bran
½ of an apple chopped into fine pieces
¼ cup raisins
Dash of crushed
A pinch of crushed cinnamon
A pinch of salt
Soy milk if desired for serving

Cooking Method
Boil water on high heat in a saucepan. Add in the Oat bran and stir while letting the water come back to boiling point, after which point you need to lower the heat on the stove and stir the pan for two more minutes while it cooks. After the two minutes cut off the heat but don't take the pan off the stove, toss in the raisins, apples and spices and stir until you can see the apple bits softening. This will take around 5 minutes. You can serve the cereal with soy milk if you like.

Banana Burrito

Serves 2

Nutritional Value: Calories: 201, Total Fat: 9.9g, Total Carbohydrates: 26.3g, Protein: 5.3g

Prep Time: 2 minutes

Cooking Time: 0 minutes

Ingredients
¼ cup natural butter
1 whole what tortilla
½ cup diced bananas
½ cup strawberries
½ cup raspberries (optional)
¼ cup raw oats
¼ cup chia seeds
¼ cup finely chopped nuts

Cooking Method
Place the tortilla on a butter paper, spread the natural butter all over it into a fine layer. Add the assortment of bananas, berries, nuts and oats and roll the tortilla into a burrito.

Quinoa

Serves 4

Nutritional Value: Calories: 338, Total Fat: 16.9g, Total Carbohydrates: 41.2g, Protein: 7.3g

Prep Time: 0 minutes

Cooking Time: 15 minutes

Ingredients
2 teaspoon vanilla extract
2 tablespoon maple syrup
1 cup crushed and toasted walnuts
1 cup fresh blueberries
1 cup raw quinoa
1 cup almond milk (unsweetened)
Salt to taste

Cooking Method
Boil the quinoa in the almond milk and add the vanilla and salt before the pan reaches boiling point. At boiling point decrease the heat to a medium flame, put on the lid and let the ingredients simmer for 13 to 14 minutes. When you see the quinoa becoming tender and chewy and the milk has been absorbed in. Dish out the quinoa and serve with an extra squirt of 2 to 4 tablespoons of almond milk on top of it then you can place the blueberries and walnuts as you like and pour some maple syrup on top. Remember to serve while hot.

Broiled Grapefruit

Serves 1

Nutritional Value: Calories: 41, Total Fat: 0.1g, Total Carbohydrates: 10.3g, Protein: 0.8g

Prep Time: 0 minutes

Cooking Time: 2-3 minutes

Ingredients
1 Grapefruit

Cooking Method
Broil the grapefruit for a couple of moments until the sugars inside the fruit are caramelized.

Healthy Oats and berry Pancakes

Serves 7

Nutritional Value: Calories: 10, Total Fat: 0.1g, Total Carbohydrates: 2.5g

Prep Time: 0 minutes

Cooking Time: 8 minutes

Ingredients
½ cup fresh blueberries
½ cup dairy free or almond milk
¾ cup flour of oats
Separate cups of 1/16 cup and 3/8 cup of Oats
½ cup of pecans or not if you are allergic
1/8 cup applesauce
½ of a banana
Pinch of cinnamon

Cooking Method
Pound the oats with the pecans. Mix all the ingredients save the blueberries in a separate bowl. When all the ingredients are well mixed you can stir in the blueberries and place in on the 325 degrees pre heated skillet. You can even shape it into anything you wish because the thickness of the batter does not spread that much. Make sure you have not placed any blueberries on the edge of the pancake as they tend to fall out when cooking. You need to cook each side for around three minutes; it will become apparent when the sides become visibly browner and thicker. Serve with the toppings of your choice.

Vegan Cornbread Waffles Topped With Pumpkin Slices

Serves 8

Nutritional Value: Calories: 387, Total Fat: 29.0g, Total Carbohydrates: 31.6g, Protein: 6.8g

Prep Time: 5 minutes

Cooking Time: 3- 5 minutes

Ingredients

1 cup water
½ teaspoon salt
2 teaspoon pumpkin pie spice
2 tablespoon olive oil
2 flax seeds
6 tablespoons ripe banana
½ cup almond meal
2/3 cup cornmeal
1 cup buckwheat flour
2 cup pumpkin puree
3 cups almond milk
A dash of shredded cloves
A dash of nutmeg
Caramelized cinnamon apples (for topping)

Cooking Method

Mix all ingredients before adding water and flour to them. Check the consistency until the desired thickness is reached and the batter is thick. Spread a thick layer of batter in the waffle maker, do not assume that the batter will settle and spread if you leave it. Cook each waffle from 3 to 5 minutes.

Fruity Oatmeal

Serves 2

Nutritional Value: Calories: 281, Total Fat: 3.6g, Total Carbohydrates: 58.0g, Protein: 7.8g

Prep Time: 0 minutes

Cooking Time: 2-3 minutes

Ingredients

1 cup rolled oats
1 teaspoon cinnamon
1 cup water
1 sliced banana
4 tablespoons soy milk, vanilla flavored
Blackberries (for topping)
Sliced bananas (for topping)
Strawberries cut in half (for topping)

Cooking Method

Combine together the cinnamon and oats in a bowl before adding water and stirring. Remember to use a microwave safe bowl so that you can cook the oats in the microwave for a minute. Toss in the banana slices into the bowl and do not forget to stir nicely before cooking the ingredients for one more minute. When you take out the bowl you can pour in the soy milk and use the berries and pieces of bananas for topping.

Banana Smoothie

Serves 1

Nutritional Value: Calories: 720, Total Fat: 30.3g, Total Carbohydrates: 41.9g, Protein: 13.2g

Prep Time: 2 minutes

Cooking Time: 0 minutes

Ingredients
1 cup water
1 banana sliced
½ cup vanilla
¼ cup quinoa
¼ cup raw walnuts
2 teaspoon flax oil
1 medjool date without the seed
1 vanilla bean flesh
¾ teaspoon crushed cinnamon
A dash of allspice

Cooking Method
Toss all ingredients into the blender and blend till smooth. If you cannot find vanilla flesh you can use ½ teaspoon of pure vanilla extract.

Apple Pie Shake

Serves 2

Nutritional Value: Calories: 238, Total Fat: 5.3g, Total Carbohydrates: 48.1g, Protein: 4.5g

Prep Time: 2 minutes

Cooking Time: 0 minutes

Ingredients

1 cup water/ almond milk
5 ice cubes
½ avocado diced
2 sliced apples
4 cups spinach
1 cucumber
Dash of crushed nutmeg
½ teaspoon vanilla extract/ maple extract
1 teaspoon crushed cinnamon
2 tablespoons walnuts
1 cup apple juice

Cooking Method
Toss all ingredients into the blender and blend until smooth.

The Total Vegan Smoothie

Serves 2

Nutritional Value: Calories: 22, Total Fat: 0.4g, Total Carbohydrates: 3.4g, Protein: 2.6g

Prep Time: 2 minutes

Cooking Time: 0 minutes

Ingredients

2 sliced cucumbers
An inch of fresh ginger root
4 cups diced honey dew melon
2 teaspoon lemon juice
6 cups uncooked spinach
2 cups organic green tea

Cooking Method
Blend all ingredients together till smooth.

Appetizers, Dips and Seasonings

Salsa

Serves 1

Nutritional Value: Calories: 76, Total Fat: 1.1g, Total Carbohydrates: 16.2g, Protein: 3.7g

Prep Time: 2 minutes

Cooking Time: 0 minutes

Ingredients

Lime
Cilantro
5-6 green onions
½ teaspoon cumin
4- 5 garlic cloves
1 teaspoon chili powder
Roma Tomatoes cut in 4 pieces

Cooking Method
Toss all ingredients in a food processor and blend. Remember not to over blend and make the dish smooth. You need to keep it chunky. Salsa can be served, on top of rice, with beans, mango, papaya and lime juice.

Crackers

Serves 3

Nutritional Value: Calories: 279, Total Fat: 10.0 g, Total Carbohydrates: 41.7 g, Protein: 5.8g

Prep Time: 5 minutes

Cooking Time: 15 minutes

Ingredients
1 ¼ cup whole wheat flour
1 teaspoon dried herbs (for seasoning)
1 teaspoon chili powder (for seasoning)
1 teaspoon garlic powder (for seasoning)
1 teaspoon onion powder (for seasoning)
A dash of salt
2 tablespoons olive oil or canola oil
2 Oz water

Cooking Method
Take first only the 1 cup of flour and ½ teaspoon of the salt and oil and put it in the food processor. Pulse the mixer a bit then add 3 tablespoons of water and turn on the processor. You can use commeal, rye or buckwheat as your whole wheat.

You need add more water as the blades pulse. The idea is to get a compact ball, you can always add more flour if you find the ball too sticky to handle even after dusting your hands. Remember to dust your workstation with flour (a piece of parchment or baking paper works too). Remember to divide the dough into portions and when you roll out the dough you need to make sure that the thickness of the dough is 1/8 of an inch.

If you are using a parchment paper you can reuse it several times for different batches. Also if you feel that the dough is too dry when you roll it, do not continue, put the entire dough back in the food processor and add more water.

Preheat the oven to 400 degrees and bake the flat dough for 10 minutes or you can extend to 15 if they are not yet light brown. You need to cool the circular crispy crackers and break them into pieces before serving.

Toasted Nuts

Serves 1

Nutritional Value: Calories: 85, Total Fat: 0.7 g, Total Carbohydrates: 20.9g, Protein: 1.1 g

Prep Time: 0 minutes

Cooking Time: 15 minutes

Ingredients
Handful of walnuts
A handful of almonds
A handful of cashews
A handful of any other nuts of your choice
A sprinkle of unsweetened raisins

Cooking Method
Take a baking sheet and place an assortment of all the nuts you have chosen on the sheet. Preheat the oven to 400 degrees and bake the nuts for 15 minutes or lesser if you see the nuts get slightly brown. Serve with unsweetened raisins after cooling the nuts.

Fire Cracker Green Beans Snack

Serves 1

Nutritional Value: Calories: 241, Total Fat: 27.2 g, Total Carbohydrates: 0.1 g, Protein: 0.0 g

Prep Time: 0 minutes

Cooking Time: 5 minutes

Ingredients

2 tablespoons oil
1 pound trimmed green beans
¼ teaspoon salt
3 crushed garlic cloves
A dash of red pepper flakes

Cooking Method

Pour some oil in a frying pan and turn the heat on medium high flame. Toss in the salt and green beans. Stir the beans for around 2-3 minutes as they cook. After that you can add the crushed garlic and red pepper flakes and cook for 1 last minute before it is ready to serve.

Guacamole

Serves 2
Nutritional Value: Calories: 435, Total Carbohydrates: 22.8g, Total Fats: 39.5g, Protein: 5.0g

Prep Time: 0 minutes

Cooking Time: 2 minutes

Ingredients
2 avocados
Juice of 1 lime
2 garlic cloves
1 Roma Tomato
Pinch of salt
¼ of Jalapeno

Cooking Method
Toss all ingredients in a food processor and blend till smooth. You can enjoy this as a dip with vegetables, mushrooms or beans.

Gazpacho

Serves 2
Nutritional Value: Calories: 140, Total Carbohydrates: 17.4g, Total Fats: 7.9g, Protein: 3.1g

Prep Time: 1 minutes

Cooking Time: 5 minutes

Ingredients
1 tablespoon lemon juice
1 tablespoon extra virgin olive oil
½ green bell pepper
½ teaspoon ground cumin seed
1 cup vegetable stock
½ zucchini sliced
1 cucumber
½ teaspoon sea salt
½ teaspoon cayenne pepper
3 tomatoes cut in 4 pieces
½ red onion
2 small garlic cloves, ground
Handful of parsley
Handful of chives
Handful of basil

Cooking Method
First blend the pepper, garlic, zucchini, onion, cucumbers and tomatoes. Make sure you do not blend till smooth, stop the processor when the mixture still looks a bit chunky. Transfer in the cumin, cayenne, salt, oil, lemon juice and herbs and blend a few more rounds before pouring in the vegetable stock. Blend completely and pour out the mixture in a large bowl. You need to refrigerate the Gazpacho at least one hour before serving.

Mediterranean Hummus with Crackers

Serves 4

Nutritional Value: Calories: 218, Total Carbohydrates: 36.4g, Total Fats: 2.9g, Protein: 13.0g

Prep Time: 0 minutes

Cooking Time: 5 minutes

Ingredients
½ teaspoon ground cumin
1 small garlic clove, ground
1 tablespoon lemon juice
Pinch of salt and cayenne pepper
1 tablespoon tahini
8 Oz black beans (with liquid)

Cooking Method
Add the black beans (save the liquid), garlic clove, salt and cayenne, cumin, tahini and lemon juice into the blender and blend till the mixture is smooth. Start adding the bean's liquid until you think the mixture has become consistent enough. Pulse through and serve with crackers.

Fried Sauce

Serves 3
Nutritional Value: Calories: 53, Total Carbohydrates: 11.1g, Total Fats: 0.6g, Protein: 3.5g

Prep Time: 0 minutes

Cooking Time: 7 minutes

Ingredients
1 cup sliced broccoli
Dash of oregano
Pinch of sea salt
1 clove garlic
1 cup thinly sliced mushrooms
5 Roma tomatoes cut in small cubic pieces

Cooking Method
Take a pan and prepare cooking the garlic, onion and oregano on low heat. Toss in all the vegetables and cook thoroughly. Finally transfer it to a small bowl for serving.

Salty Seasoning

Serves 3

Nutritional Value: Calories: 72, Total Carbohydrates: 6.6g, Total Fats: 5.5g, Protein: 1.4g

Prep Time: 0 minutes

Cooking Time: 5 minutes

Ingredients
1 tablespoon garlic powder
2 teaspoon black pepper
2 teaspoon oregano flakes
1 ½ tablespoon paprika
2 teaspoon thyme
1 tablespoon salt
2 teaspoon cayenne pepper
A tablespoon of extra virgin olive oil

Cooking Method
Use a whisking utensils to beat all the ingredients together, In the end add in some extra virgin olive oil and whisk that in thoroughly too. Transfer the seasoning from bowl into a glass bottle or airtight container.

Veggie Soup

Serves 4
Nutritional Value: Calories: 57, Total Carbohydrates: 12.2g, Total Fats: 0.3g, Protein: 2.4g

Prep Time: 0 minute

Cooking Time: 15 minutes

Ingredients

1 ½ cup seeded Roma tomatoes, cut up in small equal pieces
2 cups sliced carrots
2 cups sliced celery
2 cups chopped mushrooms
40 Ounces of Vegetable stalk
1 ½ cup finely chopped onion
2 cups of sliced red, green or yellow pepper
¾ cup Barley

Cooking Method

Take a suitable soup cooking spot, Use only ¼ cup of the vegetable stalk to first pour in the pot follow with all the vegetables and cook them until they are entirely tender. Toss the spices in the pot and stir them in with the rest of the cooked ingredients. Pour in the rest of the vegetable stalk and boil the contents. Toss in the Barley and Boil for around 15 minutes or less if Barley is tender.

Lunch

Veggie Tacos

Serves 7
Nutritional Value: Calories: 79, Total Carbohydrates: 15,9g, Total Fats: 1.1g, Protein: 2.1g

Prep Time: 5 minutes

Cooking Time: 10 minutes

Ingredients
Grape Seed oil
Salsa
8 Oz mashed potatoes
7 tortillas

Cooking Method
Preheat Oven to 350 degrees. Spread a bit of oil on each tortilla on both sides. Put around two tablespoons of mash potatoes in each tortilla and roll it half (or any way you want as long as it does not open) and align the tacos on a baking sheet. Bake for ten minutes until they are all crispy. Serve with Salsa.

Fresh Fruit Salad

Serves 1
Nutritional Value: Calories: 40, Total Carbohydrates: 7.0g, Total Fats: 0.5g, Protein: 3.6g

Prep Time: 0 minutes

Cooking Time: 5 minutes

Ingredients
4 peeled kiwifruits cut in semi circle shapes
¼ cup chopped red onion
4 cups spinach leaves
½ can pineapple slices (with juice)

Cooking Method
Put all ingredients in a bowl and top with the pineapple juice. Toss the contents gently with salad utensils.

Corn and Bean Salad

Serves 2
Nutritional Value: Calories: 284, Total Carbohydrates: 25.6g, Total Fats: 19.2g, Protein: 7.4g

Prep Time: 0 minutes

Cooking Time: 5 minutes

Ingredients

1 tablespoon lime juice
3 teaspoons mashed cilantro
½ tomato diced
¼ cup minced red onion
1 tablespoon extra virgin olive oil
1 Oz black beans
1 cup finely sliced red cabbage
¼ cup pine nuts
¾ cup kernel corns

Cooking Method

First cook the pine nuts in a pan on medium –low flame until you see them going lightly brown. Take a separate bowl to beat the lime, cilantro, salt and pepper together in. Eventually add the corn, cabbage, tomato, onion, beans and the cooked pine nuts. Refrigerate and do not forget to sprinkle ground salt and pepper before serving.

Brown Rice with Veggies

Serves 2
Nutritional Value: Calories: 617, Total Carbohydrates: 122.4g, Total Fats: 8.1g, Protein: 15.4g

Prep Time: 0 minutes

Cooking Time: 15 minutes

Ingredients
1 ½ cup cooked brown rice
¼ Oz sesame oil
4 teaspoons ground ginger
2 cups finely chopped broccoli
1 ½ finely sliced green onions
½ can of water chestnuts (get the sliced ones if you can)
¾ cup unfrozen peas
1 sliced carrot
2 cups finely chopped spinach
¼ pound mashed green beans
¼ cup toasted almond chunks
1 ground garlic clove

Cooking Method
Heat a dry and deep frying pan on a medium flame for 1 minute. Then add the sesame oil and keep the heat on for another minute. Toss in first the ginger and onions, cook these for 5 minutes. At this point toss in the carrots, garlic, green beans and broccoli and fry these for around 6 minutes. Add the chopped spinach and after a moment throw in the peas, almonds, brown rice and chestnuts. Serve hot.

Stir Fried Brown Rice

Serves 2
Nutritional Value: Calories: 582, Total Carbohydrates: 116.3g, Total Fats: 7.6g, Protein: 12.5g

Prep Time: 0 minutes

Cooking Time: 10 minutes

Ingredients
½ tablespoon olive oil
1 cup finely sliced broccoli
½ cup sliced carrots
¼ cup finely chopped onion
1 ½ tablespoon Liquid aminos
4 teaspoons natural orange juice
1 ground garlic clove
½ teaspoon ground ginger
1 ½ cup cooked brown rice
½ Oz finely chopped green onion

Cooking Method
Heat a frying pan over a medium flame and sprinkle in the olive oil. Toss the onions, carrots and broccoli into the pan and cook until the vegetables get soft. Eventually raise the flame to medium- high and put in the rest of the ingredients. Cook for around 5 minutes. Serve while hot.

Whole Food Tortillas

Serves 4
Nutritional Value: Calories: 157, Total Carbohydrates: 32.9g, Total Fats: 0.6g, Protein: 4.1g

Prep Time: 0 minutes

Cooking Time: 5 minutes

Ingredients
2 cup risen whole wheat dough
¼ cup brown rice
½ teaspoon salt
½ cup water

Cooking Method
Separate the dough into 4 portions and roll the portions into around 8 inch circles. Sprinkle olive oil in a pan and turn on the medium-low heat. Cook the rolled tortillas for only a minute. Turn the tortillas the other side and cook them for around 2 minutes until you see it bubbling up.

Rice Cakes with Avocado

Serves 2
Nutritional Value: Calories: 479, Total Carbohydrates: 55.1g, Total Fats: 26.2g, Protein: 11.6g

Prep Time: 5 minutes

Cooking Time: 7 minutes

Ingredients
1 sliced Avocado
¾ cup cooked wild rice
1 tablespoon ground oats
1 tablespoon sliced onions
¼ Oz olive oil
2 teaspoons tahini
2 teaspoons ground parsley
Salt to taste

Cooking Method
Save the Avocado and combine all ingredients thoroughly in a mixing bowl. Take a saucepan and heat it on a medium- high flame. To make one rice cake you need ½ of the mixture. Even out the portions on the pan with a spatula, try to make it circular. You need to cook 5 minutes on one side and 2 on the other. Before serving, use avocado slices as a topping on the cake. Serve warm.

Fried Beans

Serves 3
Nutritional Value: Calories: 232, Total Carbohydrates: 42.0g, Total Fats: 0.8g, Protein: 14.3g

Prep Time: 0 minutes

Cooking Time: 15minutes

Ingredients
7 Oz pinto beans
¼ teaspoon garlic powder
Dash of onion powder
Sliced green onions (without the heads)

Cooking Method
Cook the beans in a skillet over a medium flame for around 5 minutes. Use your stirring utensil to crush them until they are coarsely smooth. Cut the flame to low and let it cook for an additional 10 minutes. At this point, sprinkle over the sliced green onions and stir them in. Serve while hot.

Quick Lunch Spinach Smoothie

Serves 2

Nutritional Value: Calories: 306, Total Carbohydrates: 77.8g, Total Fats: 1.2g, Protein: 5.2g

Prep Time: 0 minutes

Cooking Time: 4 minutes

Ingredients

2 cups coconut water
1 ½ cups ice cubes
2 cups pineapple chunks
4 cups baby spinach
4 sliced bananas

Cooking Method

Toss all ingredients in a blender and blend until smooth.

Red Beans with Tasty Creole Seasoning

Serves 4
Nutritional Value: Calories: 378, Total Carbohydrates: 72.1g, Total Fats: 3.1g, Protein: 16.5g

Prep Time: 0 minutes

Cooking Time: 10 minutes

Ingredients

1 cup cooked brown rice
¼ cup chopped celery
8 Oz red kidney beans
1 teaspoon olive oil
¼ cup sliced red onion
2 tablespoons water
¼ cup finely sliced green pepper
1 teaspoon Creole seasoning

Cooking Method

Over a medium flame heat the extra virgin olive oil in a pan and toss in first the celery, onions and peppers. Cook until they become soft. That would take 4 minutes. Add in the Creole Seasoning and water. Stir them in and follow by mixing in the rice and kidney beans. Cook for another 5 minutes. Serve hot.

Dinner

Rice and Roasted flavor Sauce

Serves 8
Nutritional Value: Calories: 378, Total Carbohydrates: 76.6g, Total Fats: 3.9g, Protein: 6.8g

Prep Time: 0 minutes

Cooking Time: 15minutes

Ingredients
4 cups cooked rice
2 cups red pepper sauce
4 cups Chinese Long beans, sliced
1 Oz olive oil
½ cup water
2 Oz liquid Amino
2 cups sliced onion rings

Cooking Method
Pour in the oil in a large pan, heated on a medium flame. Toss in the long beans and onions, cook these for 4 minutes. Add the aminos, water and rice. Stir these three ingredients in. Stop cooking when the water is mostly absorbed. Heat the Red pepper sauce in a separate pan on a low flame. When heated top the sauce on each serving of rice.

Steamy Flatbread

Serves 8

Nutritional Value: Calories: 303, Total Carbohydrates: 54.9g, Total Fats: 6.0g, Protein: 11.4g

Prep Time: 0 minutes

Cooking Time: 15 minutes

Ingredients

5 cups risen whole grain flour dough
2 tablespoon extra virgin olive oil
1 teaspoon dried basil
1 teaspoon garlic powder
1 teaspoon dried parsley

Cooking Method

Use the entire dough and roll it out into a quarter of an inch layer on a baking sheet. Mix Olive oil, Basil and garlic powder across in a small bowl and make tiny holes alla cross the dough (preferably with a fork). Brush the olive oil mixture on top of the poked dough. Remember to make cuts, not all the way through in the dough before you put it in the oven. The cuts should indicate the portion size. Bake for 15 minutes in a 400 degrees preheated oven. Cut into portions before serving.

4 Minute Nutritious Veggies

Serves 2

Nutritional Value: Calories: 125, Total Carbohydrates: 9.1g, Total Fats: 10.1g, Protein: 2.0g

Prep Time: 4 minutes

Cooking Time: 0 minutes

Ingredients

2 equally sliced tomatoes
½ avocado peeled and sliced
Pinch of finely chopped basil
Pinch of salt

Cooking Method

Use 4 Avocado slices and place them on a couple of Tomato slices. Sprinkle them with basil and salt.

Fried Black Beans with Avocado Garnish

Serves 3

Nutritional Value: Calories: 438, Total Carbohydrates: 77.1g, Total Fats: 5.2g, Protein: 24.8g

Prep Time: 0 minutes

Cooking Time: 15 minutes

Ingredients

1 Oz olive oil
1 cup chopped onion
30 Oz black beans
30 Oz diced tomatoes
1 cup corn kernels
½ cup red pepper, diced
½ cup green pepper, diced
2 garlic cloves
2 Oz lime juice
1 teaspoon cumin
½ teaspoon salt
¼ teaspoons crushed black pepper
Avocado slices

Cooking Method

Heat the onions in the oil on a medium low flame. The onions need to become crisp y and dark. At this point you should toss in the peppers, corn, tomatoes, garlic, lime, beans, cumin and salt and pepper. Let the ingredients cook for approximately 15 minutes. Cut off the heat and t the Avocado as a topping before serving.

Sweet Potatoes and Onions

Serves 2

Nutritional Value: Calories: 279, Total Carbohydrates: 37.9g, Total Fats: 13.5g, Protein: 3.6g

Prep Time: 1 minute

Cooking Time: 14 minutes

Ingredients

1 Oz olive oil
½ cup diced onion
¾ pounds sweet potato

Cooking Method

Cut the sweet potatoes in chunky strips and combine them with the onions in a dry bowl. Take a medium pan and pour only half of the oil in it to heat over a medium- low flame. Toss in the entire potato/ onion mixture and stir it rotating it so that it absorbs the oil. Remember to stop stirring for 7 minutes as the food cooks. Flip the food on the other side and let that side cook for the same amount of time. Serve while hot.

Tofu Flavored Rice

Serves 4

Nutritional Value: Calories: 332, Total Carbohydrates: 55.5g, Total Fats: 8.9g, Protein: 11.1g

Prep Time: 0 minutes

Cooking Time: 15 minutes

Ingredients
½ Oz olive oil
1 tofu marinade (saved from marinated tofu)
½ Oz olive oil
1 cup finely diced onions
2 cups sliced broccoli
1 cup finely sliced carrots
1 ground garlic clove
½ tablespoon tahini
1 teaspoon crushed ginger
2 Oz pineapple juice
1 ½ cup cooked wild rice
¼ cup tasted walnut chunks
1 teaspoon sesame seeds

Cooking Method
Use a large pan to heat the oil in over a medium heat. First toss in only the onions till they become soft, then add the ginger, garlic, carrots, broccoli and the tofu marinade. Cover the pan with a lid and let the vegetables simmer for 8 minutes. You may remove the lid a couple of times to stir. At the end just sprinkle in the pineapple juice and walnuts and add the rice. Cook until you see the juice is all absorbed. At this point cut off the heat and top each serving with sesame seeds.

Bean Burger Subs

Serves 2
Nutritional Value: Calories: 380, Total Carbohydrates: 60.0g, Total Fats: 5.8g, Protein: 22.7g

Prep Time: 5 minutes

Cooking Time: 10 minutes

Ingredients
1 teaspoon olive oil
½ Oz diced onion
½ cup black beans
½ cup northern beans
½ Oz flaxseed meal
½ teaspoon garlic powder
Pinch of cumin
Pinch of salt

Cooking Method
Use a large skillet to fry the onions in olive oil until they become soft. Remove the onions but do not discard the oil or the pan. Take only ¾ of your entire bean ingredient for this meal and use a mashing utensil to crush the beans in a mixing dish. Add the fried onions into this dish and toss in the salt, cumin, flaxseed meal and garlic powder.

Turn on the heat back under the pan on a medium flame. Divide the bean mixture into portions and cook each portion by flattening it with a spatula to make them look like a patty. You will need to cook each side of the patty for around 5 minutes. Serve them stuffed in a burger or a sandwich.

Tropical Wild Rice

Serves 3
Nutritional Value: Calories: 361, Total Carbohydrates: 68.6g, Total Fats: 4.3g, Protein: 15.2g

Prep Time: 0 minutes

Cooking Time: 11 minutes

Ingredients
¼ Oz olive oil
¼ cup diced onion
1 small ground garlic clove
4 Oz Pineapple slices
½ Oz liquid aminos
2 teaspoons lime juice
½ cup chopped carrots
½ cup crushed snow peas
½ cup finely chopped zucchini
¼ cup roasted bell peppers
¼ cup black beans
¼ cup chickpeas
1 cup cooked wild rice

Cooking Method
Cook the onions in olive oil over a medium flame. When you see the onions becoming soft toss in the garlic and stir it for 1 minute while it cooks. Add the Aminos, lime juice and Pineapple juice. Follow with throwing in the chickpeas, snow peas, carrots, beans, red peppers and zucchini. At this point you should raise the flame to medium high and let it simmer for around 4 more minutes. Toss in the rice and pineapple and fry them until they are cooked entirely. Serve while hot.

Stuffed Bells

Serves 4

Nutritional Value: Calories: 68, Total Carbohydrates: 5.9g, Total Fats: 4.3g, Protein: 2.7g

Prep Time: 0 minutes

Cooking Time: 5 minutes

Ingredients
2 bell peppers sliced
½ cup hummus
1/2 cup chopped tomato
¼ cup sliced black olives
2 teaspoon finely diced avocado
Pinch of sunflower seeds

Cooking Method
Take a small bowl and combine olives, tomatoes and hummus thoroughly. Take two tablespoons of the hummus mixture and stuff them in the halved bell peppers. Top the filling with sunflower seeds and avocado.

Roasted Asparagus

Serves 3

Nutritional Value: Calories: 38, Total Carbohydrates: 4.6g, Total Fats: 1.9g, Protein: 2.5 g

Prep Time: 0 minutes

Cooking Time: 15 minutes

Ingredients

Salt to taste
¼ tablespoon olive oil
Pinch of tarragon
Pinch of garlic powder
½ pound trimmed asparagus

Cooking Method

Brush a baking dish with extra virgin olive oil and cut the asparagus into spears. Align them on the dish and first brush the food with oil and in a separate bowl mix salt, garlic powder and tarragon well. Coat the asparagus entirely with this mixture. Roast the Asparagus for 15 minutes in a 450 degrees preheated oven.

Made in the USA
Las Vegas, NV
15 July 2023

74768471R00037